JEFF HAPPI

Fitness guidebook for men

Unlock Your Best Body and Achieve Peak Performance: A Comprehensive Guide to Fitness for Men

Copyright © 2024 by Jeff Happi

All rights reserved. No part of this publication may be reproduced, stored or transmitted in any form or by any means, electronic, mechanical, photocopying, recording, scanning, or otherwise without written permission from the publisher. It is illegal to copy this book, post it to a website, or distribute it by any other means without permission.

Jeff Happi asserts the moral right to be identified as the author of this work.

Jeff Happi has no responsibility for the persistence or accuracy of URLs for external or third-party Internet Websites referred to in this publication and does not guarantee that any content on such Websites is, or will remain, accurate or appropriate.

Designations used by companies to distinguish their products are often claimed as trademarks. All brand names and product names used in this book and on its cover are trade names, service marks, trademarks and registered trademarks of their respective owners. The publishers and the book are not associated with any product or vendor mentioned in this book. None of the companies referenced within the book have endorsed the book.

First edition

This book was professionally typeset on Reedsy.
Find out more at reedsy.com

Contents

1

Introduction

Fitness is more than a trend - it's a lifestyle. It's a way of living that prioritizes physical health and well being. And while the world of fitness may seem overwhelming at first, it's important to remember that it's never too late to start your fitness journey. Whether you're looking to lose weight, build muscle, or simply maintain a healthy lifestyle, there are countless options available to help you get started. In this introduction, we'll explore the basics of fitness, why it matters, and how you can make it a part of your daily routine.

Why Fitness Matters:

Fitness is so much more than just looking good in a swimsuit. It's about improving your overall health and well being. Regular physical activity can help reduce the risk of chronic diseases like diabetes, cardiovascular disease, and certain types of cancer. It's also been shown to improve cognitive function, mood, and sleep quality.

But the benefits of fitness go beyond just physical health. Exercise and healthy habits are essential for emotional well being as well. Regular exercise can help reduce stress levels, anxiety, and symptoms of depression. It's one of the best ways to promote mental health and well being.

About Fitness:

At its core, fitness is about movement. Physical activity is the foundation of your fitness journey, and it's essential for maintaining good cardiovascular health, building muscle, and improving overall physical fitness.

Strength training is a great way to build muscle, increase strength, and support joint health. It involves lifting weights, using resistance bands, or performing bodyweight exercises like push ups, squats, and lunges. Starting with lighter weights and working your way up gradually is essential to prevent injury.

Cardiovascular exercise, or cardio, is also crucial for optimal fitness. Cardio workouts get your heart rate up, improve cardiovascular health, and help with weight loss. Running, cycling, swimming, and dancing are all great forms of cardio that can be done indoors or outdoors.

Nutrition is another important component of your fitness journey. A balanced diet that includes plenty of fruits and vegetables, lean proteins, whole grains, and healthy fats is critical for maintaining good health. Stay away from processed foods, sugary drinks, and foods high in saturated fats.

Rest is also an essential part of your fitness journey. Giving your body the rest it needs to recover between workouts is critical to preventing injury and burnout. Getting enough quality sleep, staying hydrated, and taking rest days are important components in any fitness routine. We will talk more about it later.

One of the biggest hurdles to starting a fitness journey is getting started. Many people are intimidated by the gym or don't know where to begin. But it's important to remember that there are many options available to help you get started.

One of the best ways to get started is by finding a workout buddy or partner. Having someone to exercise with can be motivating and help keep you accountable. It can also make workouts more enjoyable and help you stay on track.

Group fitness classes are also a great option for beginners. Classes like yoga, Pilates, and spinning are great for those who are new to exercise or prefer working out in a group setting. They provide structure and guidance, making it easier to get started.

Hiring a personal trainer is another option for those who are new to fitness or looking to take their workouts to the next level. Personal trainers can help create a tailored workout plan that's specific to your individual needs. They can also help with proper form and technique, which is important for preventing injury.

Injuries and Setbacks:

Injuries and setbacks are a normal part of any fitness journey. They can be frustrating, but they don't have to derail your progress. When it comes to injuries, prevention is key. Proper warm up and cool-down, choosing appropriate workout gear, and seeking medical attention for injuries are all important steps in preventing injuries.

If you do experience an injury, it's important to listen to your body and seek medical attention if necessary. Depending on the severity of the injury, modifying your workout routine or switching to low-impact exercises may be necessary.

Setbacks like weight loss plateaus or lack of motivation are also normal parts of any fitness journey. It's important to stay committed to your goals and remember why you started your fitness journey in the first place. Celebrating small victories along the way and engaging in self-care techniques like meditation, deep breathing, and quality sleep can help you get back on track.

Whether you're just beginning your fitness journey or looking to take your workouts to the next level, it's important to remember that fitness is about finding a way to move your body, fuel it with the right nutrition, and take care of your mental well being. The journey towards fitness can be challenging, but with the right mindset, tools, and strategies, anyone can achieve their goals. Remember to celebrate small victories along the way, take care of your body, and stay committed to your goals. With perseverance and dedication, you can achieve optimal fitness and live a happier, healthier life.

2

CHAPTER 1

Why You Haven't Achieved Your Fitness Goals Yet

If you're reading this book, chances are you've struggled to achieve your fitness goals in the past. But why is that? Here are some common reasons why people struggle to make progress in their fitness journey:

1. **Lack of motivation**: Sometimes it can be tough to find the motivation to work out or eat healthily, especially if you're feeling stressed or overwhelmed. Try to find activities that you enjoy and that make you feel good, and remember that being active is a great way to relieve stress.

2. **Lack of accountability**: Holding yourself accountable for your actions can be tough, especially if you're used to making excuses or procrastinating. Consider partnering up with a friend or hiring a personal trainer to help keep you on track.

3. **Unrealistic expectations**: When it comes to fitness, it's important

to set realistic expectations for yourself. Remember that progress takes time, and it's okay to start small. Celebrate small victories along the way and be patient with yourself.

4. Lack of knowledge: If you're new to fitness, it can be overwhelming to navigate all the different workout routines, equipment, and nutrition information out there. Consider hiring a personal trainer or taking classes to learn more about what works best for your body.

Achieving optimal fitness is a journey that requires dedication, patience, and consistency. By focusing on regular physical activity, a balanced diet, and rest and recovery, you can start to make progress towards your fitness goals. Remember to be patient with yourself, celebrate small victories along the way, and don't be afraid to ask for help when you need it. With perseverance and determination, you can achieve optimal fitness and live a happier, healthier life.

3

CHAPTER 2

Discipline & Organization are the Key

« No one saves us but ourselves. No one can and no one may. We ourselves must walk the path »
BUDDHA

When it comes to achieving your fitness goals, discipline and organization are two of the most important factors that will determine your success. Discipline means having the mental and physical fortitude to stick to your plan, even when it's tough. Organization means having the systems and structures in place to keep you on track and working efficiently.

Get Your Mind and Your Space Clean

Before you can begin to implement discipline and organization in your life, it's important to get your mind and your space clean. This means decluttering your physical environment, as well as your mental space. Here are some tips on how to achieve this:

1. Declutter Your Physical Environment:

You've probably heard the saying "a cluttered space equals a cluttered mind," and it's true. When your physical environment is cluttered and disorganized, it can make it difficult to focus and be productive. Take the time to declutter your space by getting rid of anything you don't need and organizing what's left. This will not only help you feel more productive but also more relaxed.

2. Clean Out Your Mental Space:

Your mental space is just as important as your physical environment. If you're constantly racing thoughts and worries, it can be tough to focus on the task at hand. Try journaling or meditation to help clear your mind and declutter your thoughts. By creating a clean mental space, you'll be better equipped to stay disciplined and organized.

3. Create a Schedule:

Another way to stay organized is to create a schedule for your day. This could be as simple as writing down a to-do list for the day or creating a more detailed daily planner. By having a plan in place, you'll be less likely to waste precious time and more likely to stay productive.

Getting Started

Now that you've created a clean mental and physical space and have a plan in place, it's time to get started. Here are some tips for staying disciplined and organized as you work towards your fitness goals:

1. Stay Focused:

It's easy to get distracted by social media, email, or other distractions throughout the day. To stay focused, consider breaking up your day into 30-minute or hour-long increments, dedicating specific blocks of time to certain tasks. This will not only help you stay on task but also break your day down into more manageable chunks.

2. Stay Accountable:

Hold yourself accountable for your progress by tracking your progress towards your goals. This could be through a journal, a spreadsheet, or a digital tool like a habit tracker. By tracking your progress, you'll be better equipped to see where you're making progress and where you need to improve.

3. Celebrate Your Victories:

It's important to celebrate your victories, even the small ones. By taking the time to recognize your progress and celebrate your successes, you'll be more motivated to keep pushing forward towards your goals.

Finding Your Motivation

When it comes to staying disciplined and organized in your fitness journey, finding motivation is key. Here are some tips for finding and maintaining motivation:

1. Find Your Why:

Identifying the reason behind your fitness journey is essential. Knowing why you're making these changes will help you stay on track and motivated. Maybe it's to improve your health, feel better about yourself, or set a good example for your family. Whatever your reason, make it a priority and use it as a driving force to keep pushing forward.

2. Connect with Others:

Connecting with others who share your goals is a great way to stay motivated. Surround yourself with people who support your journey, whether it's a workout partner, a social media community, or a fitness group. When you have others encouraging you along the way, it's easier to stay accountable and motivated.

3. Set Realistic Goals:

Setting realistic, achievable goals is important to maintaining motivation. If you set goals that are too lofty or unrealistic, it can be easy to get discouraged. Instead, break your goals down into smaller, achievable milestones. Celebrate each victory along the way, no matter how small, and use it as fuel to keep going.

The Power of Habits

Another way to stay disciplined and organized in your fitness journey is to create healthy habits. Habits are powerful tools that can help you stick to your plan without relying on sheer willpower. Here are some tips for creating healthy habits:

1. Start Small:

Don't try to overhaul your entire life in one day. Instead, start small by implementing one healthy habit at a time. This could be something as simple as drinking more water or going for a walk after dinner. By starting small and building momentum, you'll be more likely to create lasting habits.

2. Make It a Routine:

Once you've identified a healthy habit you'd like to create, make it a routine. Whether it's scheduling a workout at the same time every day or meal-prepping on Sundays, creating a routine will help you establish a healthy habit.

3. Stay Consistent:

Consistency is key when it comes to creating healthy habits. Try to stick to your new habit for at least 21 days to create a lasting change. Once you've established one new habit, you can start working on another.

In conclusion, discipline and organization are essential in achieving your fitness goals. By creating a clean mental and physical space, staying focused on your goals, and implementing healthy habits, you'll be well on your way to achieving success. Remember to stay motivated, celebrate your victories, and don't be afraid to ask for help along the way. With perseverance, patience, and consistency, you can achieve your fitness goals and live a happier, healthier life.

« I'm no prophet. My job is making windows where there were once walls»
MICHEL FOUCAULT

4

Chapter 3

Know Your Body: The Importance of Training Every Muscle Group

When it comes to achieving fitness success, it's easy to get caught up in focusing on one particular area of the body, like building bigger biceps or getting stronger abs. However, the key to achieving optimal fitness is to train every muscle group in the body. A balanced and consistent training program that incorporates exercises for the abdominals, back, shoulders, legs, arms, and chest is essential. This chapter will explore the importance of training each muscle group and provide exercises to strengthen them.

ABS

The abdominal muscles are often referred to as the "core" of the body. Training the abdominals is crucial for maintaining proper posture, balance, and stability. Strengthening the abs can also help prevent lower back pain. Here are some exercises to strengthen the abdominals:

1. Plank: The classic plank exercise targets the transverse abdominals, the deep muscles responsible for stabilizing the body. To perform a plank, start in a push-up position and lower onto your forearms. Keep your body straight and hold for as long as you can.

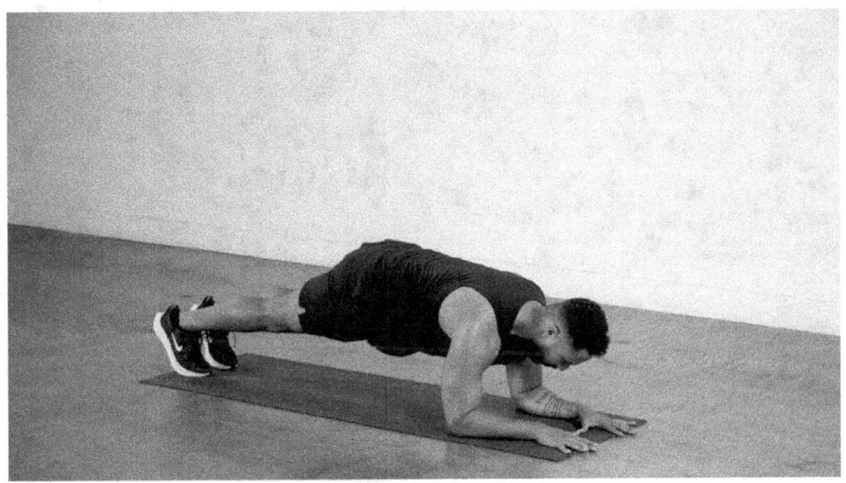

2. Russian twist: This exercise works the rectus abdominis, the muscles responsible for creating the "six-pack." Sit on the floor with your knees bent and feet flat on the ground. Lean back slightly and twist to one side, tapping your hand on the ground. Repeat on the other side.

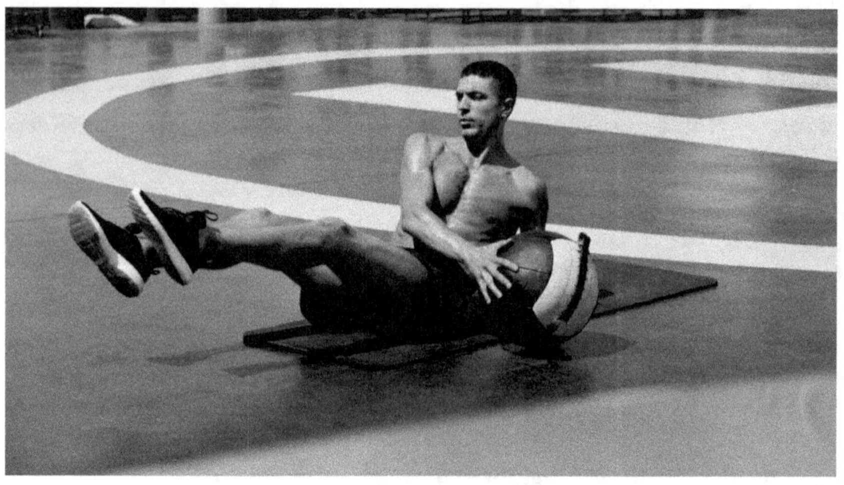

3. Leg raises: This exercise targets the lower abdominals. Lie on your back with your hands under your hips for support. Lift your legs straight up off the ground until they are perpendicular to the floor. Slowly lower your legs back down and repeat.

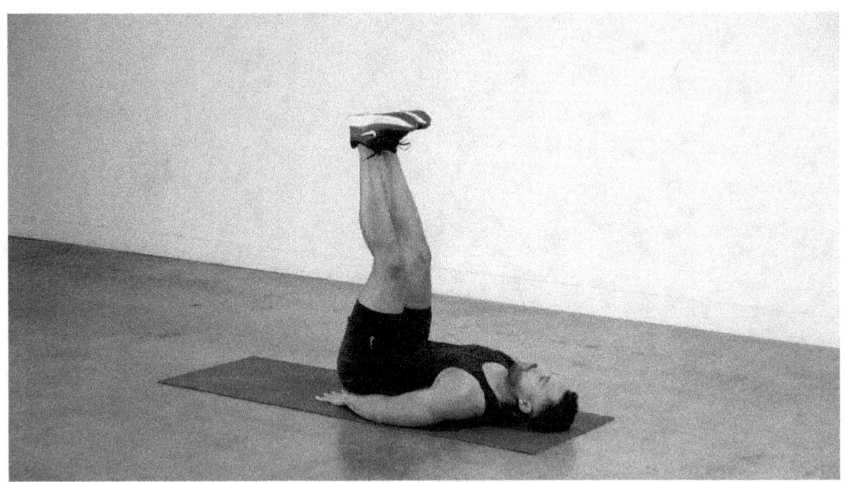

BACK

The muscles of the back are important for posture, stability, and overall body strength. By strengthening the back muscles, you can also reduce your risk of injury. Here are some exercises to strengthen the back:

1. Pull-ups: Pull-ups are an excellent exercise for targeting the back muscles, particularly the latissimus dorsi. To perform a pull-up, grip a pull-up bar with your palms facing away from you and your hands shoulder-width apart. Pull yourself up until your chin is above the bar and release back down.

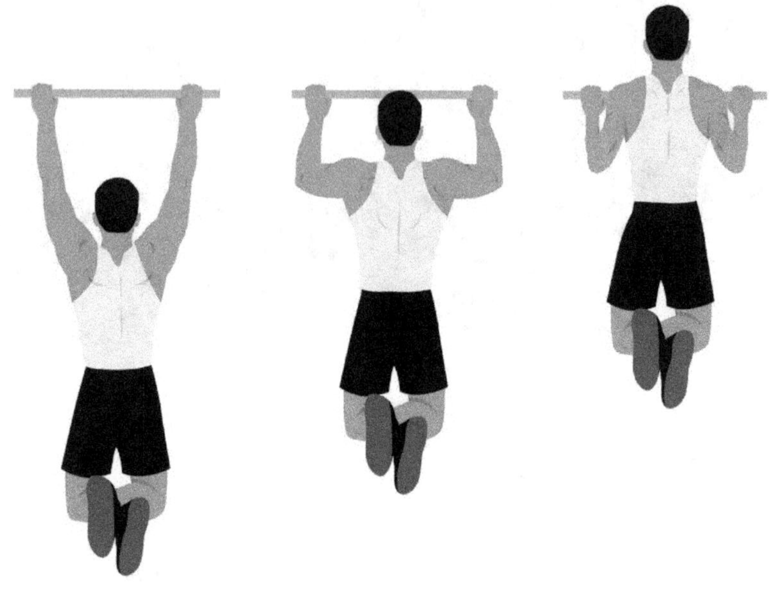

2. Bent-over rows: This exercise works the rhomboids and trapezius muscles in the upper back. With a dumbbell in each hand, bend your knees slightly and hinge forward at the hips. Pull the dumbbells up to your chest and release back down.

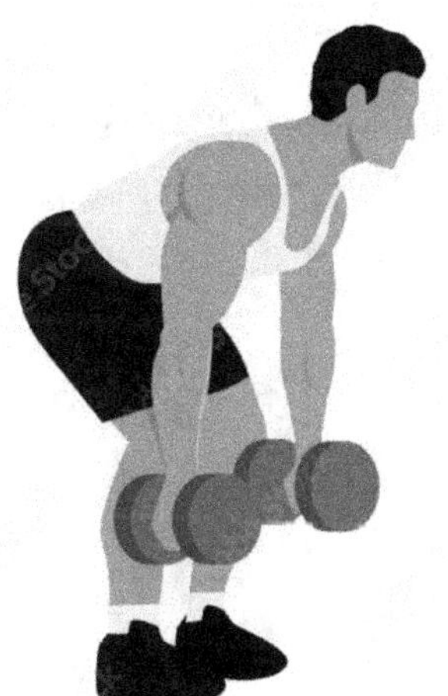 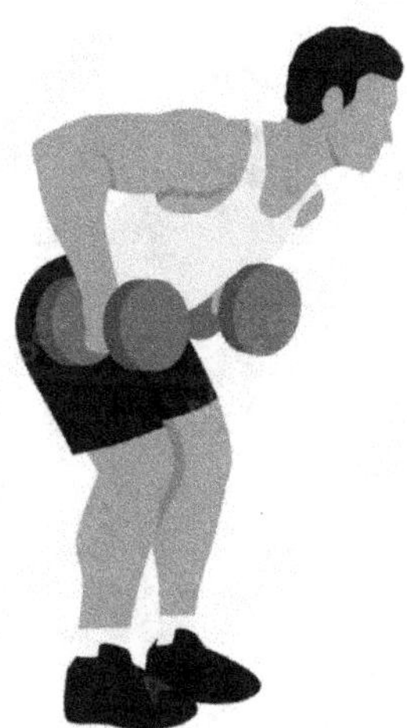

3. Superman: This exercise targets the erector spinae muscles in the lower back. Lie face down on the floor with your arms and legs extended. Lift your arms, legs, and chest off the ground and hold for a few seconds before releasing.

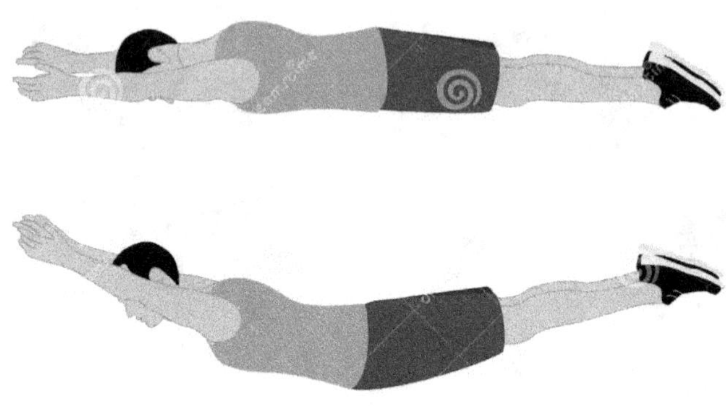

SHOULDERS

The shoulder muscles are important for overhead movements and general upper-body strength. By strengthening the shoulders, you can also improve your posture and relieve neck pain. Here are some exercises to strengthen the shoulders:

1. Shoulder press: The shoulder press works the deltoid muscles in the shoulders. Hold a dumbbell in each hand and raise your arms up to shoulder height. Extend your arms straight up until they are overhead and then release back down.

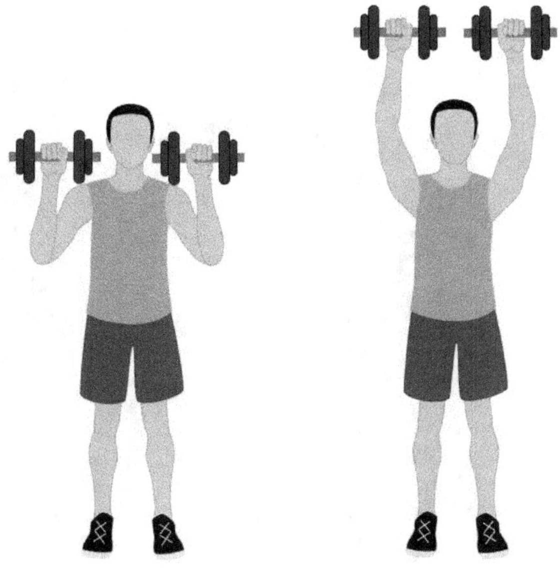

2. Lateral raises: This exercise targets the middle deltoid muscles. Hold a dumbbell in each hand and lift your arms out to the sides until they are shoulder-height. Slowly release back down.

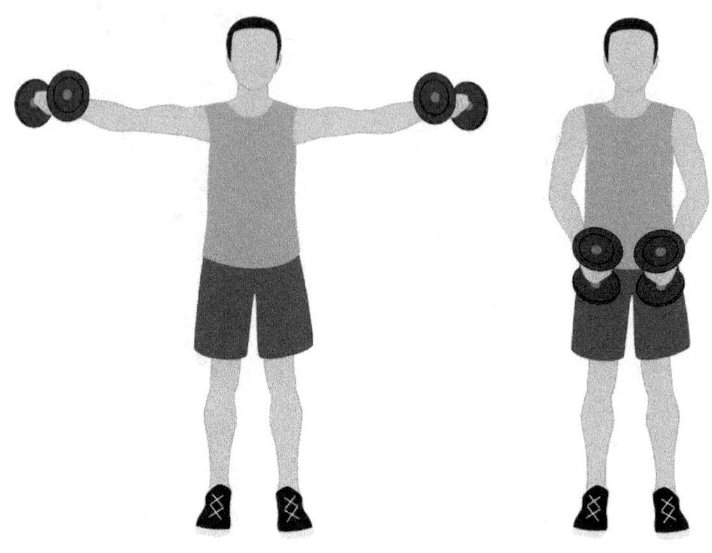

3. Rear delt flyes: This exercise targets the rear deltoid muscles. Hold a dumbbell in each hand and hinge forward at the hips, keeping your back straight. Lift your arms up and out to the sides until they are parallel to the ground and then release back down.

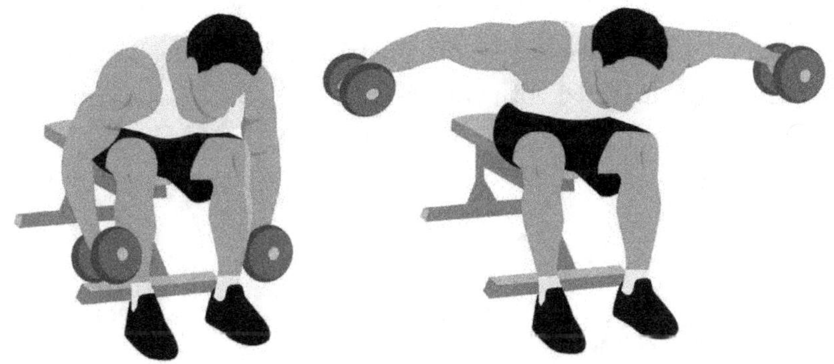

LEGS

< Don't skip legs days> Here is why:

The leg muscles are the largest muscles in the body and are responsible for many functional movements like walking, running, and jumping. By strengthening the legs, you can improve your overall athletic performance and tone your lower body. Here are some exercises to strengthen the legs:

1. Squats: The classic squat exercise targets the quadriceps, hamstrings, and gluteus maximus. Stand with your feet shoulder-width apart and squat down, keeping your back straight and your knees behind your toes.

2. Lunges: This exercise targets the quadriceps, hamstrings, and gluteus maximus. Step forward with your right leg and bend your knee until your thigh is parallel to the ground. Return to standing and repeat on the other side.

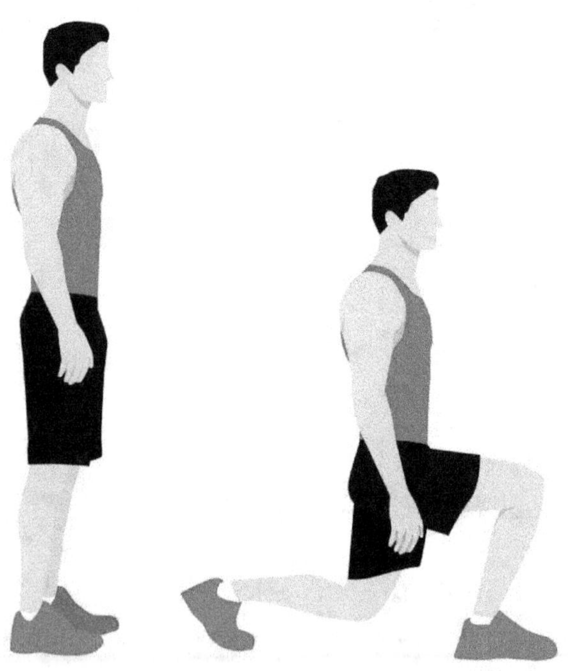

3. Deadlifts: This exercise targets the hamstrings, gluteus maximus, and lower back. With a barbell in front of you, bend down to grip the bar with an overhand grip. Stand up, keeping your back straight and the bar close to your body, and then release back down.

ARMS

The arm muscles are essential for many upper body movements like lifting, pulling and pushing. By strengthening the arm muscles, you can improve your overall strength and tone your upper body. Here are some exercises to strengthen the arms:

1. Bicep curls: The classic bicep curl targets the biceps muscles in the front of the arm. Hold a dumbbell in each hand and curl the weights towards your shoulders, keeping your elbows tucked in.

2. Tricep dips: This exercise targets the triceps muscles in the back of the arm. Place your hands on a bench behind you with your fingers pointing towards your body. Lower your body down towards the ground and then push back up.

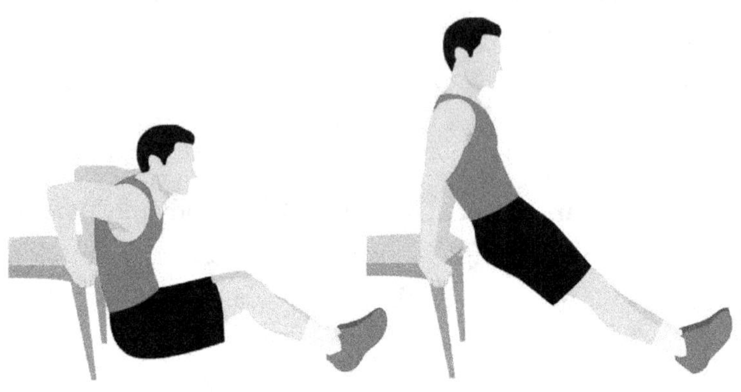

3. Hammer curls: This exercise targets the brachialis muscles in the upper arm. Hold a dumbbell in each hand with your palms facing towards your body. Curl the weights up towards your shoulders and release back down.

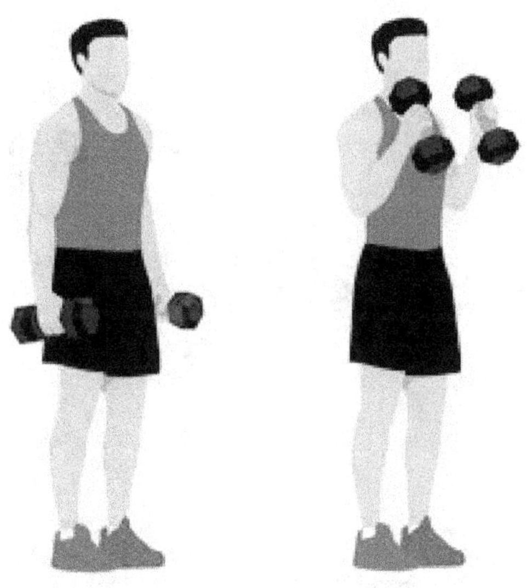

CHEST

The chest muscles are important for many upper body movements like pushing and pulling. By strengthening the chest muscles, you can also improve your posture and overall upper body strength. Here are some exercises to strengthen the chest:

1. Push-ups: The classic push-up targets the pectoralis major muscles in the chest. Start in a plank position with your hands shoulder-width apart. Lower your body down towards the ground, keeping your elbows tucked in, and push back up.

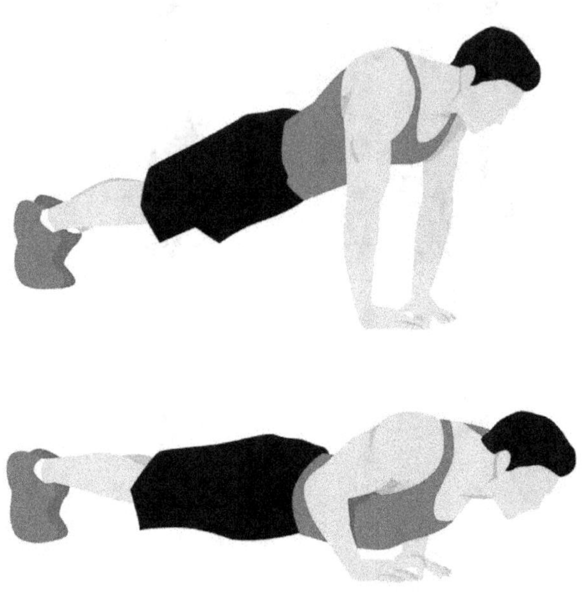

2. Chest press: This exercise can be done with dumbbells or a barbell and targets the pectoralis major muscles in the chest. Lie on a bench with your feet on the ground and lift the weights up to your chest. Extend your arms straight up and then release back down.

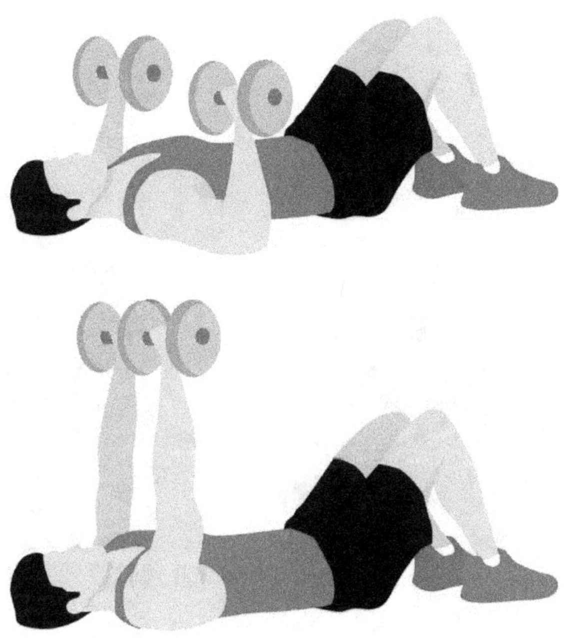

3. **Chest flyes**: This exercise targets the pectoralis major muscles in the chest. Lie on a bench with your feet on the ground and hold a dumbbell in each hand. Open your arms out to the sides until they are parallel to the ground and then release back down.

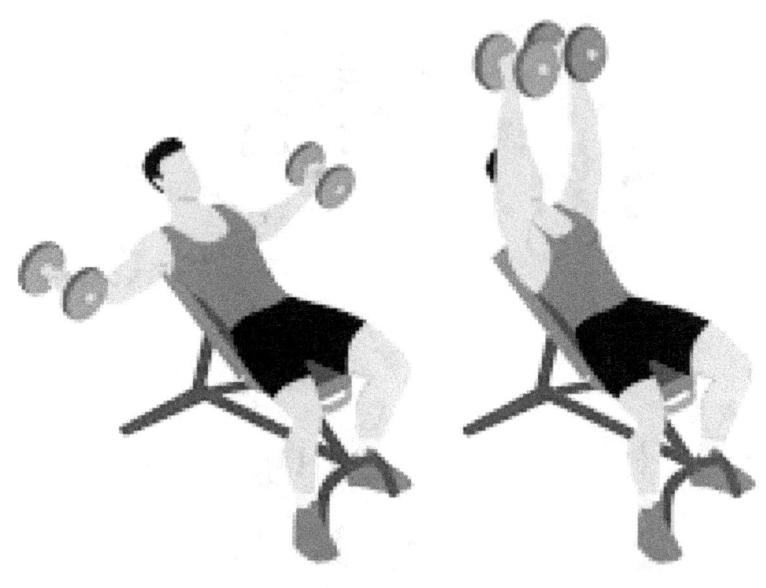

What you need to understand is training all of the muscle groups in the body is essential for achieving optimal fitness. By incorporating exercises for the abdominals, back, shoulders, legs, arms, and chest, you can improve your overall strength, posture and support functional movements. Remember to perform each exercise with proper form, stay consistent, and gradually increase weight and reps to see results.

5

CHAPTER 4

Cardio

When it comes to achieving optimal fitness, incorporating cardio into your exercise routine is essential. Cardiovascular exercise, or cardio for short, helps strengthen your heart and lungs, improve overall endurance, and burn calories. But with so many different types of cardio exercises out there, how do you know which one is right for you? Read on to discover the benefits of cardio exercise and some popular options to try.

Benefits of Cardio Exercise

1. Heart health: Cardio exercise helps to strengthen the heart muscle, improves circulation, and reduces the risk of heart disease.

2. Weight loss: Cardio is an excellent way to burn calories and lose weight.

3. Stress relief: Cardio exercise releases endorphins, which are "feel-good" hormones that help reduce stress and anxiety.

4. Improved energy levels: Regular cardio exercise can boost energy levels, reduce fatigue, and improve overall mood.

Types of Cardio Exercise

1. Running: Running is a popular form of cardio exercise that can be done outdoors or on a treadmill. It provides a high-intensity workout that burns a lot of calories and improves overall fitness levels.

2. Cycling: Cycling is a low-impact form of cardio that's easy on the joints. It can be done outdoors or on a stationary bike and provides great cardiovascular benefits.

3. Swimming: Swimming is a full-body workout that provides a low-impact form of cardio exercise. It also strengthens the muscles, improves endurance, and burns calories.

4. Jumping rope: Jumping rope is a fun and high-intensity form of cardio that can be done almost anywhere. It burns calories quickly and is great for improving coordination and overall fitness levels.

5. Dancing: Dancing is a fun and creative way to get your cardio exercise in. It burns a lot of calories, improves coordination, and is a great stress reliever.

6

CHAPTER 5

Nutrition Matters

No matter how much you exercise, proper nutrition is essential for achieving optimal fitness. Eating a well-balanced and varied diet that provides all the nutrients your body needs is key. Here are some important considerations when it comes to nutrition and fitness.

1. **Macronutrients:** The three macronutrients - carbohydrates, proteins, and fats - provide energy and are necessary for overall health and fitness. Eating a variety of foods that provide all three macronutrients in the right proportions is important.

2. **Micronutrients:** Vitamins and minerals are essential for maintaining good health and proper body function. Eating a varied and colorful diet that includes a variety of fruits and vegetables is key to getting all the micronutrients your body needs.

3. **Hydration**: Water is critical for good health and fitness. Staying

hydrated helps lubricate the joints, regulate body temperature, and support proper digestion. Aim to drink at least eight glasses of water a day, and more if you're exercising.

4. Meal timing: The timing of your meals can also impact your fitness levels. Eating a balanced meal before exercise can provide the energy needed to perform well, while consuming a meal after exercise can help with recovery and muscle building.

5. Supplements: While it's best to get most of your nutrients from food, certain supplements like protein powder, fish oil, and multivitamins can be helpful in ensuring you get all the nutrients your body needs for optimal fitness.

7

CHAPTER 6

Sleep Quality

Sleep is often overlooked when it comes to achieving optimal fitness, but it's just as important as exercise and proper nutrition. Proper sleep quality provides critical benefits for physical and mental health. Here are some tips for improving sleep quality and reaping the benefits.

1. Sleep duration: Aim to get seven to nine hours of quality sleep each night. Consistently sleeping less than this can increase the risk of chronic diseases and negatively impact overall fitness levels.

2. Sleep environment: Create a sleep-friendly environment by keeping the room dark, cool, and quiet. Investing in a comfortable mattress and pillows can also help improve sleep quality.

3. Sleep hygiene: Establish a regular sleep routine by going to bed and waking up at the same time each day. Avoid electronics, caffeine, and alcohol for several hours before bedtime, as these can interfere with sleep quality.

4. Relaxation techniques: Practicing relaxation techniques like meditation, deep breathing, or yoga can also help improve sleep quality by reducing stress and promoting relaxation.

5. Seek help: If you have persistent sleep difficulties like insomnia or sleep apnea, seek medical help. These conditions can negatively impact overall fitness and require treatment to improve sleep quality.

In conclusion, achieving optimal fitness involves more than just exercise. Incorporating cardio exercise, proper nutrition, and quality sleep into your routine is essential. With consistency and dedication, you can achieve optimal fitness and enjoy all the physical and mental benefits that come with it.

8

Conclusion

Achieving optimal fitness is a journey that requires dedication, patience, and consistency. By focusing on regular physical activity, a balanced diet, rest and recovery, cardio exercise, proper nutrition, and quality sleep, you can start to make progress towards your fitness goals. Remember to be patient with yourself, celebrate small victories along the way, and don't be afraid to ask for help when you need it.

When it comes to physical activity, consistency is key. Finding activities that you enjoy and can stick to is essential for building a regular exercise routine. Whether you prefer jogging, cycling, weight lifting or yoga, it's important to prioritize physical activity in your life. Regular exercise can help improve physical health, reduce stress, and promote mental well being.

Incorporating cardio into your exercise routine is essential for achieving optimal fitness. Cardiovascular exercise helps to strengthen your heart and lungs, improve overall endurance, and burn calories. Running, cycling, swimming, jumping rope, and dancing are popular forms of cardio exercise that provide great cardiovascular benefits. Cardio exercise can help reduce the risk of heart disease, lower blood pressure, and improve cholesterol levels.

Proper nutrition is also essential for achieving optimal fitness. Eating a well-balanced and varied diet that provides all the nutrients your body needs is key. Macronutrients like carbohydrates, proteins, and fats, are necessary for overall health and fitness. Eating a variety of foods that provide all three macronutrients in the right proportions is important. Vitamins and minerals are essential for maintaining good health and proper body function. Eating a varied and colorful diet that includes a variety of fruits and vegetables is key to getting all the micronutrients your body needs.

Staying hydrated is important for maintaining good health and fitness. Drinking at least eight glasses of water a day, and more if you're exercising, helps lubricate the joints, regulate body temperature, and support proper digestion.

Above all, rest and recovery are crucial for achieving optimal fitness. Getting enough quality sleep, taking rest days, and staying hydrated are all essential for allowing your body to recover from physical activity. Poor sleep quality, on the other hand, can negatively impact all aspects of health and fitness, from physical performance to cognitive function and emotional well being.

If you're struggling to achieve your fitness goals, you're not alone. Lack of motivation, accountability, unrealistic expectations, or lack of knowledge can all be reasons why you may be struggling to make progress. Remember to be patient with yourself, set realistic expectations, and celebrate small victories along the way. Don't be afraid to ask for help when needed, whether that means hiring a personal trainer or finding an accountability partner.

Achieving optimal fitness is not just about looking good - it's about feeling good both physically and mentally. Regular exercise, proper nutrition, rest, and recovery all contribute to good physical and mental health. By prioritizing these elements, you can enjoy increased energy, reduced stress levels, and improved overall well being.

In conclusion, achieving optimal fitness is a holistic approach that takes into account all aspects of your well being. Combining regular physical activity, cardio exercise, balanced nutrition, adequate rest, hydration, and quality sleep, is crucial for optimizing your overall health and well being. Be kind to yourself, stay motivated, and commit to long-term consistency to achieve long-lasting physical and mental health benefits. Remember that small changes in habits can add up to big results over time. By staying dedicated and committed to the journey, you can achieve optimal fitness and experience the benefits of good health and well being.

If you found this book helpful, I would be very appreciative if you left a favorable review on Amazon!

www.ingramcontent.com/pod-product-compliance
Lightning Source LLC
Chambersburg PA
CBHW050753250726

48662CB00005B/2187